# TOOLS FOR CAREGIVERS

it rea
ith a

- **F&P LEVEL:** D
- **WORD COUNT:** 35

**CURRICULUM CONNECTIONS:**
community, community helpers

## Skills to Teach

- **HIGH-FREQUENCY WORDS:** a, get, has, her, I, is, it, my, she, takes, this
- **CONTENT WORDS:** chair, checks, dentist, good, look, new, nice, office, teeth, tools, toothbrush, X-rays
- **PUNCTUATION:** exclamation points, periods
- **WORD STUDY:** compound word (*toothbrush*); long /a/, spelled *ai* (*chair*); long /a/, spelled *ay* (*X-rays*); long /e/, spelled *ee* (*teeth*); /oo/, spelled *ew* (*new*); /oo/, spelled *oo* (*good, tools*); /s/, spelled *c* (*office*)
- **TEXT TYPE:** factual description

## Before Reading Activities

- Read the title and give a simple statement of the main idea.
- Have students "walk" though the book and talk about what they see in the pictures.
- Introduce new vocabulary by having students predict the first letter and locate the word in the text.
- Discuss any unfamiliar concepts that are in the text.

## After Reading Activities

This book talks about some of the items we see at the dentist's office. Have students been to the dentist? What else might they see at the dentist's office? Ask them to predict the first letter of each item, and then write its name on the board, clearly pronouncing each sound as you write.

Tadpole Books are published by Jump!, 5357 Penn Avenue South, Minneapolis, MN 55419, www.jumplibrary.com

Copyright ©2021 Jump. International copyright reserved in all countries. No part of this book may be reproduced in any form without written permission from the publisher.

**Editor:** Jenna Gleisner  **Designer:** Michelle Sonnek

**Photo Credits:** Barvista/Shutterstock, cover; Adragan/Shutterstock, 1; wavebreakmedia/Shutterstock, 2tl, 2tr, 3, 8–9, 12–13; Edvard Nalbantjan/Shutterstock, 2ml, 4–5; urfin/Shutterstock, 2mr, 6–7; Kuzina Natali/Shutterstock, 2br, 10–11; Chimpinski/Shutterstock, 2bl, 14–15; Dario Sabljak/Shutterstock, 16 (chair); Suttha Burawonk/Shutterstock, 16 (X-ray); Fototocam/Shutterstock, 16 (floss); s-ts/Shutterstock, 16 (tools); Tatiana Popova/Shutterstock, 16 (toothbrush).

Library of Congress Cataloging-in-Publication Data
Names: Zimmerman, Adeline J., author.
Title: Dentist's office / Adeline J. Zimmerman.
Description: Minneapolis, MN: Tadpole Books, (2021) | Series: Around town | Includes index. | Audience: Ages 3–6
Identifiers: LCCN 2019047530 (print) | LCCN 2019047531 (ebook) | ISBN 9781645274650 (hardcover) | ISBN 9781645274667 (paperback) | ISBN 9781645274674 (ebook)
Subjects: LCSH: Dentistry—Juvenile literature. | Children—Preparation for dental care—Juvenile literature.
Classification: LCC RK63 .Z56 2021 (print) | LCC RK63 (ebook) | DDC 617.6/45—dc23
LC record available at https://lccn.loc.gov/2019047530
LC ebook record available at https://lccn.loc.gov/2019047531

# DENTIST'S OFFICE

by Adeline J. Zimmerman

## TABLE OF CONTENTS

tadpole books

# WORDS TO KNOW

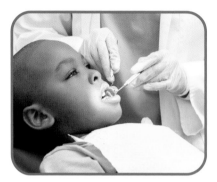

checks

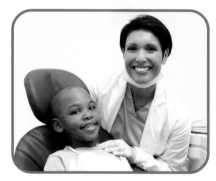

dentist

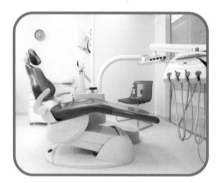

office

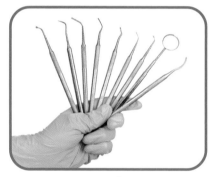

tools

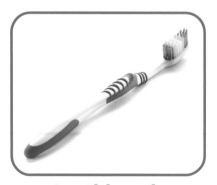

toothbrush

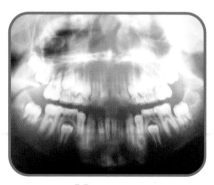

X-rays

# DENTIST'S OFFICE

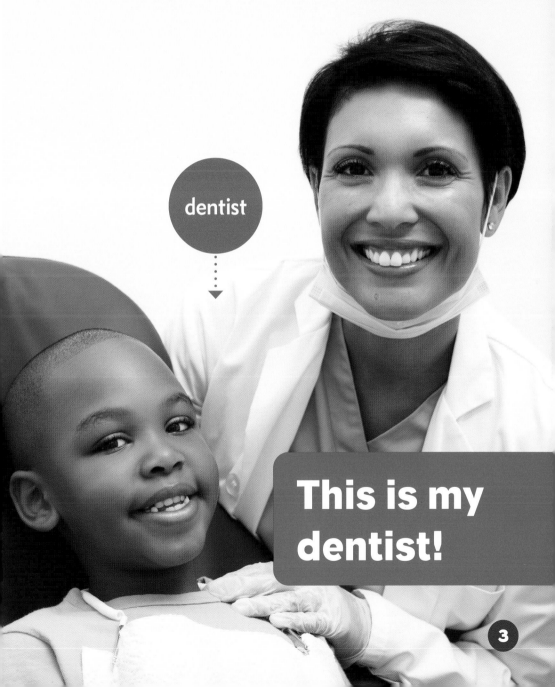

dentist

**This is my dentist!**

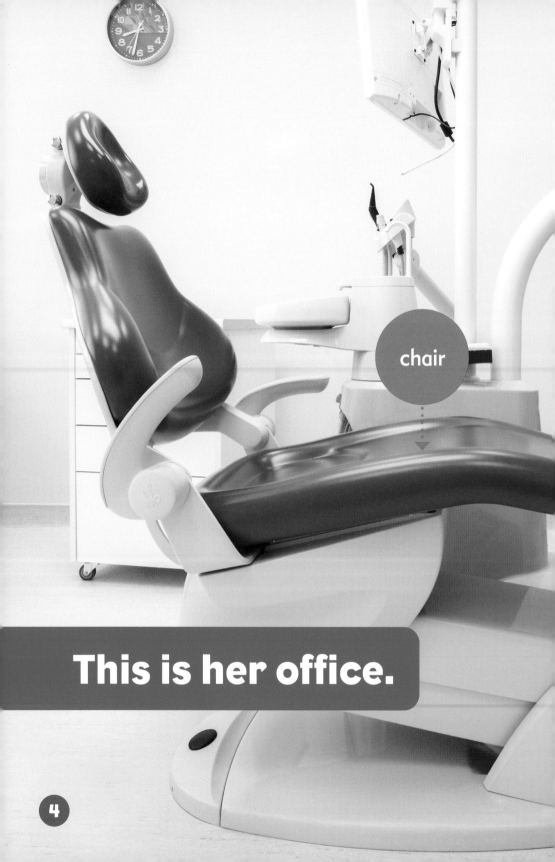

chair

**This is her office.**

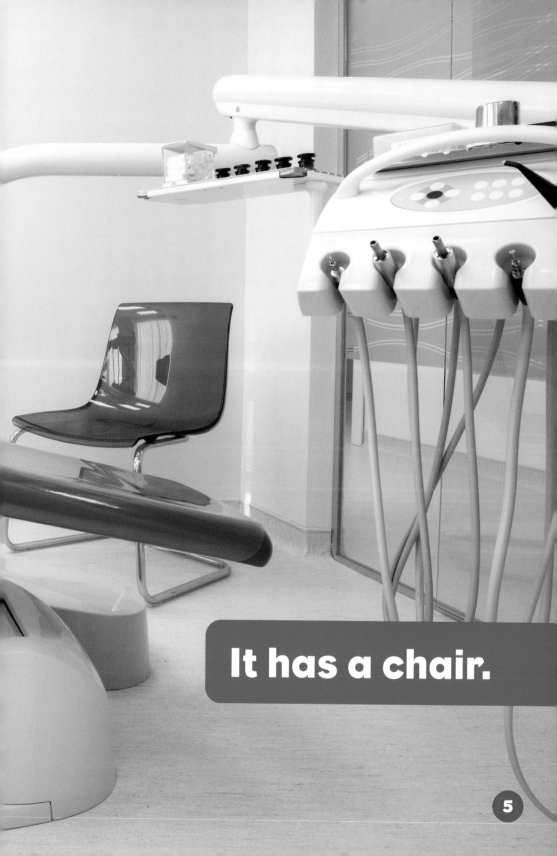

It has a chair.

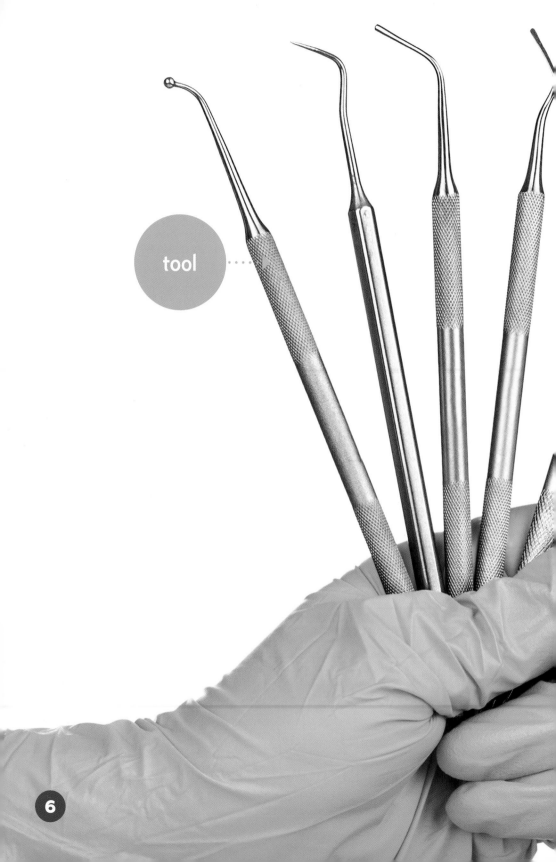

tool

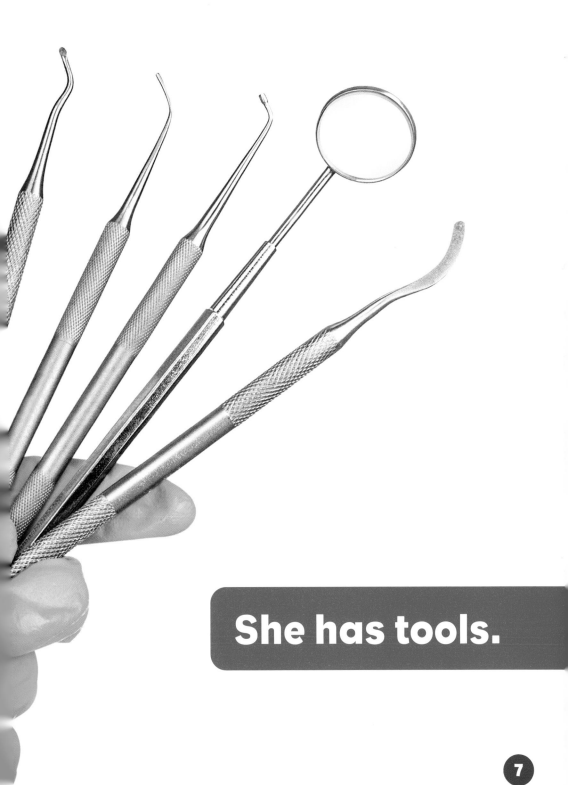

**She has tools.**

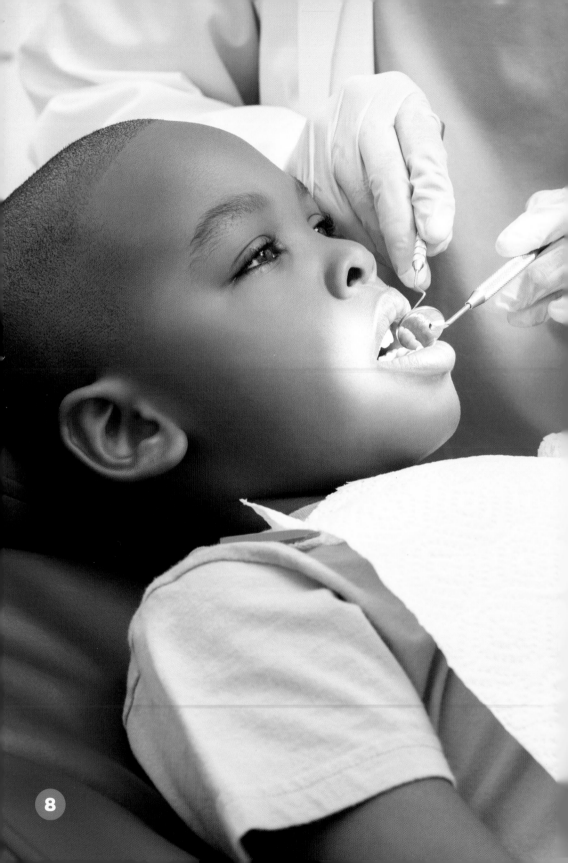

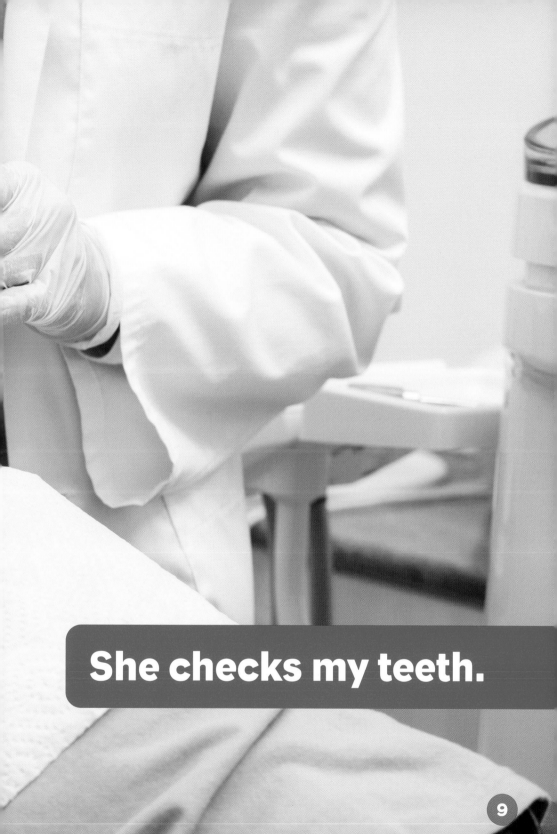

**She checks my teeth.**

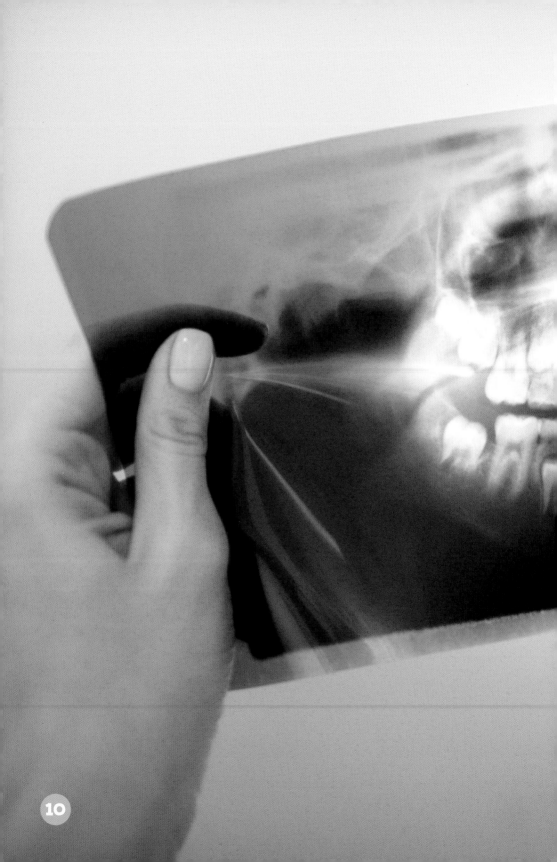

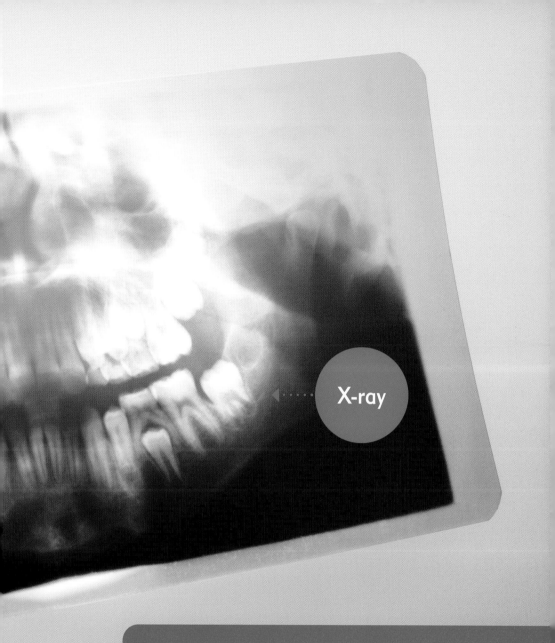

X-ray

## She takes X-rays.

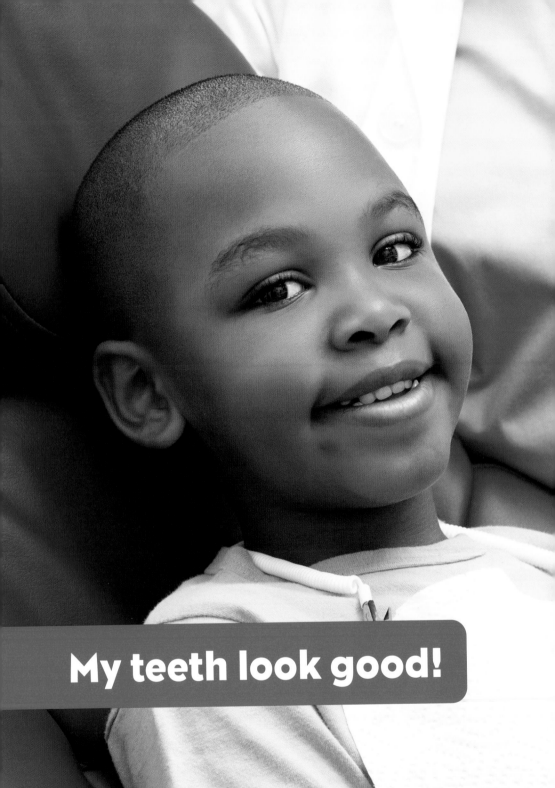

My teeth look good!

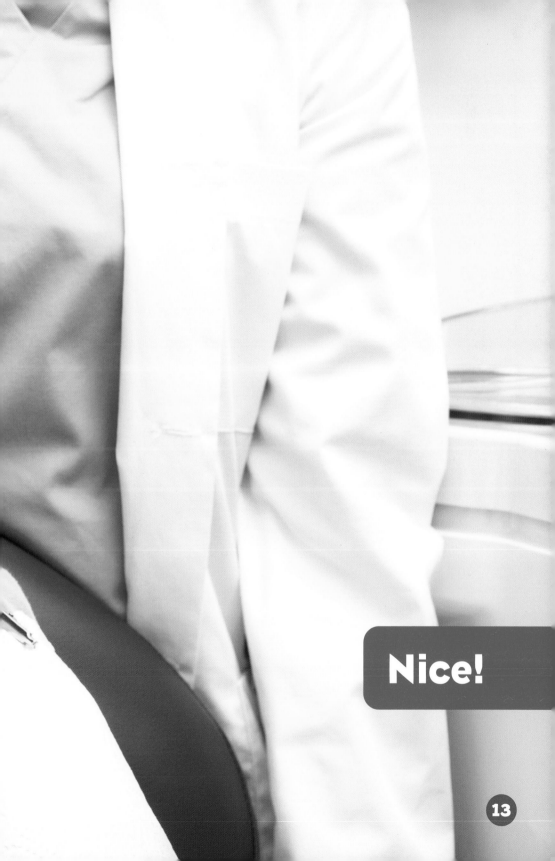

Nice!

13

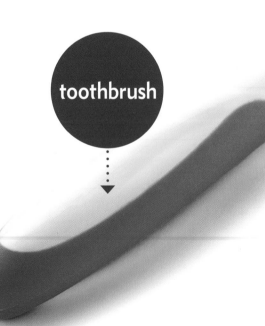

toothbrush

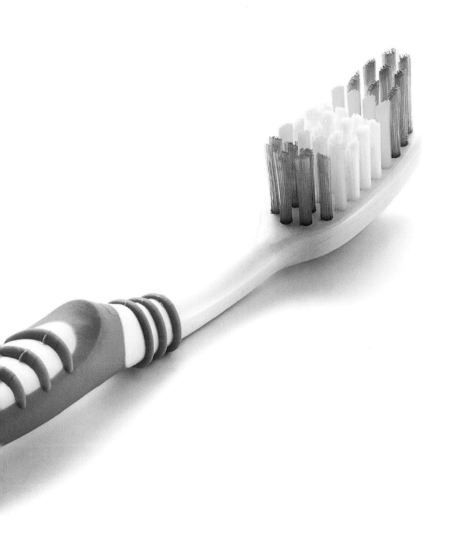

**I get a new toothbrush!**

# LET'S REVIEW!

These are all items you may see at the dentist's office. Point to and name each item.

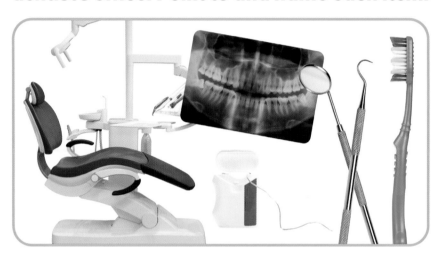

# INDEX